# A COUNTERBLAST TO TOBACCO

## A TRACT BY KING JAMES I

First Edition 1604
King James I

New Edition 2017
Edited by Tarl Warwick

A COUNTERBLAST TO TOBACCO

## **COPYRIGHT AND DISCLAIMER**

The first edition of this work is in the public domain having been written prior to 1923. This edition, with its cover art and format, is all rights reserved.

In no way may this text be construed as encouraging or condoning any harmful or illegal act. In no way may this text be construed as able to diagnose, treat, cure, or prevent any disease, injury, symptom, or condition.

# A COUNTERBLAST TO TOBACCO

# FOREWORD

King James I is perhaps best known for his tract upon demonology, entitled simply "Daemonologie" it set the stage for the worst of the burning times, as he sought to expunge the witches and heretics he saw as responsible for trying constantly to decimate his reign and the Christian religion. It is here, however, that another tract is in question; Counterblast to Tobacco, a vaguely reformist work designed simply to combat the growing use of a plant which had become popularized in use. By the time of this particular work being written, tobacco usage had skyrocketed to a level nearly as popular as alcohol, in King James' lands, as well as elsewhere in Europe, and had caused the addiction of a substantial proportion of the population to the same.

James of course reverts at times here to religious language, considering addiction to tobacco to be a sin, due to its pervasive nature and the degree of difficulty already established to exist with attempting to wean oneself off of the substance. This particular work is not so much a rigorous discourse in medical application as an opinion piece, a short text delineating James' distaste for the practice of smoking with some religious inclusions, but it is novel and of note particularly for its extremely early date of manufacture; there was no substantial anti-smoking movement prior to this work, and due to his royal status, this particular piece swayed opinion among some groups far more than it otherwise would have.

# A COUNTERBLAST TO TOBACCO

Indeed, while this tract is reformist and intellectual, it takes almost the form (especially within the introduction) as a sort of statement made by a judge rather than one of separate royal stock, with James declaring his intent to administer a just and mild purgative (after the medical sense) to the population because everyone therein, from the commoner to clergy and nobles too, has become decadent and "too wealthy" for their own good, frittering away some of that on their addiction.

It is clear that James' writing here had some degree of social impact at the time; smoking by the Victorian era became so prevalent that it found itself ingrained into the very image of rural England with its cottage gardens and quiet lifestyles, until the late pre-modern period when anti-smoking campaigns began again to proliferate; funnily there may have been fewer people smoking habitually shortly after James' tract was release, than at any other time until the 1970s or thereabouts when tobacco use began to be recognized as unhealthy.

Indeed, James here almost forms an emotional caricature; it is entirely possible to judge him for his anti-witch crusades of the similar era, but we cannot perhaps judge whether his attacks upon tobacco were derived from his personal contempt for it (perhaps some of his courtiers smoked, and it bothered him) or whether he actually cared about people enough to desire to spare them from becoming addicted to something he felt would harm their health- possibly both of these are involved with his reasoning.

This edition of Counterblast to Tobacco has been edited and rendered into modern English to the best of my ability from the original and antiquated form; care has been taken to retain all meaning associated with the original text.

Here it is interesting to note that although James holds the theory (prevailing at the time) of the humors and elements within medicine, the conclusions he has managed to reach regarding the health impacts of tobacco addiction are fundamentally correct to a great degree; specifically, he notes the nose (irritated), the lungs (poisoned), and harm to the mental faculties. He even denotes that tobacco is of a watery element, and only fiery when ignited, and then airy due to its fumes. Nasal irritation, addiction, lung problems, and mental degradation are all indeed results of excessive smoking long term and are as well documented by our modern medical establishment as they apparently were in a time before industry or even anesthesia that did not involve administering raw opium or alcohol.

# A COUNTERBLAST TO TOBACCO

## TO THE READER

As every human body (dear countrymen) however healthy it may be, is nonetheless subject, or at least naturally inclined to some sorts of diseases, or infirmities, so is there no Commonwealth, or State, however well-governed, or peaceable however it may be, that lacks the capability to contain superstition and corruption, and therefore is it no wonder, although this our country and Commonwealth, though peaceable, though wealthy, though long flourishing in both peace and wealth, be among the rest, subject to the natural problems of such a state and population. We are of all nations the people most loving and most reverently obedient to our Prince, yet are also (as time has often borne witness) too easily seduced to make Rebellion, upon very slight grounds. Our fortunate and often proved valor in wars abroad, our hearty and reverent obedience to our Princes at home, has bred us a long, and a thrice happy peace.

Our Peace has bred wealth: And peace and wealth has brought forth a general sluggishness, which makes us wallow in all sorts of idle delights, and soft delicacies, The first seeds of the subversion of all great Monarchies. Our clergy are now negligent and lazy, our nobility and gentry have become prodigal, and dedicated only to their private delights, our lawyers covet, our common-people are corrupted and curious; and generally all sorts of people more careful for their private ends, than for their

# A COUNTERBLAST TO TOBACCO

mother the Common-wealth. For the remedy to this, it is the Kings (as the proper Physician of his political body) to purge it of all those diseases, by medicines meant for the same, as by a certain mild, and yet just form of government, to maintain the public peace, and prevent all occasions of commotion, by the example of his own person and court, to make us all ashamed of our sluggish and delicate ways, and to stir us up to the practice again of all honest exercises, and to the violent specter of war. As likewise by his, and his courts humble apparel, to make us ashamed of our prodigality.

This is performed by his quick admonitions and careful overseeing of the clergy to waken them up again, to be more diligent in their offices: By the sharp trial, and severe punishment of the partial, covetous and bribing lawyers, to reform their corruptions, and generally by the example of his own person, and by the due execution of good laws, to reform and abolish, piece and piece, these old and evil grounded abuses. For this will not be *Opus unius diei,* but as every one of these diseases, must from the King receive the single cure proper for it, so are there some sorts of abuses in Common-wealths, that though they be of so base and contemptible a condition, as they are too low for the law to look on, and too mean for a King to intervene with his authority, or bend his eye upon, yet are they corruptions, as well as the greatest of them.

So is an ant an animal, as well as an elephant. So is a wren, as well as a swan, and so is a small bit of the toothache, a disease as well as the fearful plague is. But for these base sorts of corruption in Common-wealths, not only the King, or any inferior Magistrate, but *Quilibet è populo* may serve to be a

# A COUNTERBLAST TO TOBACCO

Physician, by discovering and impugning the error, and by persuading reformation thereof.

And surely in my opinion, there cannot be a more base, and yet hurtful corruption in a Country, then is the vile use (or other abuse) of taking Tobacco in this Kingdom, which has moved me, shortly to discover the abuses thereof in this following little Pamphlet.

If any think it a light argument, so it is but a toy that is bestowed upon it. And since the subject is but of smoke, I think the fume of an idle brain, may serve for a sufficient battery against so famous and feeble an enemy. If my grounds be found true, it is all I look for; but if they carry the force of persuasion with them, it is all I can wish, and more than I can expect. My only care is, that you, my dear countrymen, may rightly conceive even by this smallest trifle, of the sincerity of my meaning in great matters, never to spare any pain that may tend to the procuring of your wealth and prosperity.

## A COUNTER-BLAST TO TOBACCO

That the manifold abuses of this vile custom of tobacco use, may the better be determined, it is fit that first you enter into consideration both of the first original thereof, and likewise of the reasons of the first entry thereof into this country. For certainly as such customs, that have their first institution either from a godly, necessary, or honorable ground, and are first brought in, by the means of some worthy, virtuous, and great personage, are ever, and most justly, held in great and reverent estimation and account, by all wise, virtuous, and temperate spirits: So should it by the contrary, justly bring a great disgrace into that sort of customs, which having their original from base corruption and barbarity, doe in like sort, make their first entry into a country, by an inconsiderate and childish affectation of novelty, as is the true case of the first invention of tobacco usage, and of the first entry thereof among us. For tobacco being a common herb, which (though under many names) grows almost everywhere, was first found out by some of the barbarous Indians, to be a preservative, or antidote against the pox, a filthy disease, whereunto these barbarous people are (as all men know) very much subject, what through the uncleanly and low constitution of their bodies, and also through the intemperate heat of their climate, so that as from them was first brought into Christendom, that most detestable disease, so from them likewise was brought this use of tobacco, as a stinking and unsavory antidote, for so corrupted and execrable a malady, the stinking fumigation whereof they yet use against that disease, making so one canker or venom to destroy another.

## A COUNTERBLAST TO TOBACCO

And now good country men let us (I pray you) consider, what honor or policy can move us to imitate the barbarous and beastly manners of the wild, godless, and slavish Indians, especially in so vile and stinking a custom? Shall we disdain to imitate the manners of our neighbor, France, (having the style of the first Christian Kingdom) and that cannot endure the spirit of the Spaniards (their King being now comparable in power of Dominions to the great Emperor of Turkey). Shall we, I say, that have been so long civil and wealthy in Peace, famous and invincible in war, fortunate in both, we that have been ever able to aid any of our neighbors (but never bothered any of them with requests for aid) shall we, I say, without blushing, abase our selves so far, as to imitate these beastly Indians, slaves to the Spaniards, trash to the world, and as yet at this time aliens from the holy Covenant of God? Why do we not as well imitate them in walking naked as they do? In preferring glasses, feathers, and such toys, to gold and precious stones, as they do? Yea why do we not deny God and adore the Devil, as they do?

Now to the corrupted nature of the first use of this Tobacco, it does very well agree with the foolish and groundless first entry thereof into this Kingdom. It is not so long since the first entry of this abuse among us here, as this present age cannot yet very well remember, both the first Author, and the form of the first introduction of it among us. It was neither brought in by King, great Conqueror, nor learned Doctor of Physic.

With the report of a great discovery for a Conquest, some two or three savage men, were brought in, together with this savage custom. But the pity is, the poor, wild, barbarous men died, but that vile barbarous custom is yet alive, yea in fresh vigor: so as it seems a miracle to me, how a custom springing from so vile a ground, and brought in by a father so generally hated, should be welcomed upon so slender a warrant. For if they that first put it in practice here, had remembered for what respect it was used by them from whence it came, I am sure they would have been loath, to have taken so far the imputation of that disease upon them as they did, by using the cure thereof. For *Sanis non est opus medico*, and counter-poisons are never used, but where poison is thought to precede.

But since it is true, that various customs slightly grounded, and with no better warrant entered in a Commonwealth, may yet in the use of them thereafter, prove both necessary and profitable; it is therefore next to be examined, if there be not a full sympathy and true proportion, between the base ground and foolish entry, and the loathsome, and hurtful use of this stinking antidote.

I am now therefore heartily to pray you to consider, first upon what false and erroneous grounds you have first built the general good liking thereof; and next, what sins towards God, and foolish vanities before the world you commit, in the detestable use of it.

As for these deceitful grounds, that have especially moved you to take a good and great conceit thereof, I shall content myself to examine here only four of the principals of them; two founded upon the theories of a deceptive appearance of reason, and two of them upon the mistaken practice of general experience.

# A COUNTERBLAST TO TOBACCO

First, it is thought by you a sure Aphorism in the physics, that the brains of all men, being naturally cold and wet, all dry and hot things should be good for them; of which nature this stinking fumigation is, and therefore of good use to them. Of this argument, both the proposition and assumption are false, and so the conclusion cannot but be void of itself. For as to the proposition, that because the brains are cold and moist, therefore things that are hot and dry are best for them, it is an inept consequence: For man being compounded of the four complexions (whose fathers are the four elements) although there be a mixture of them all in all the parts of his body, yet must the varied parts of our microcosm or little world within ourselves, be more inclined to variability, some to one, some to another complexion, according to the diversity of their uses, that of these discords a perfect harmony may be made up for the maintenance of the whole body.

The application then of a thing of a contrary nature, to any of these parts is to interrupt them of their due function, and by consequence hurtful to the health of the whole body. As if a man, because the Liver is hot (as the fountain of blood) and as it were an oven to the stomach, would therefore apply and wear close upon his Liver and stomach a cake of lead; he might within a very short time (I hope) be sustained very well and inexpensively at a hospital, beside the clearing of his conscience from that deadly sin of gluttony. And as if, because the Heart is full of vital spirits, and in perpetual motion, a man would therefore lay a heavy pound stone on his breast, for staying and holding down that wanton palpitation, I doubt not but his breast would be more bruised with the weight thereof, then the heart would be comforted with such a disagreeable and contrary cure.

# A COUNTERBLAST TO TOBACCO

And even so is it with the brains. For if a man, because the Brains is cold and humid, would therefore use inwardly by smells, or outwardly by application, things of hot and dry qualities, all the gain that he could make thereof would only be to put himself in a great haste towards madness, by over-regulating his body, the coldness and moistness of our brain being the only ordinary means that procure our sleep and rest.

Indeed I do not deny, but when it falls out that any of these, or any part of our bodies grow to be distempered, and to tend to an extremity, beyond the compass of natures temperate mixture, that in that case cures of contrary qualities, to the intemperate inclination of that part, being wisely prepared and discreetly ministered, may be both necessary and helpful for strengthening and assisting Nature in the expulsion of her enemies; for this is the true definition of all profitable Physic.

But first these Cures ought not to be used, but where there is need of them, the contrary whereof, is daily practiced in this general use of tobacco by all sorts and complexions of people.

And next, I deny the minor of this argument, as I have already said, in regard that this tobacco, is not simply of a hot and dry quality; but rather has also a certain venomous faculty joined with the heat thereof, which makes it have an antipathy against nature, as can be determined by its hateful smell. For the nose being the proper Organ and convoy of the sense of smelling to the brain, which is the only fountain of that sense, serves always for an infallible witness, whether that odor which we smell, be healthful or hurtful to the brain (except when it happens that the sense itself is corrupted and abused through some infirmity, and distemper in the brain.) And that the scent thereof cannot have a drying quality, it needs no further probation, then that it is a smoke, all smoke and vapor, being of itself humid, as drawing near to the nature of the air, and easy to be resolved again into water, whereof there needs no other proof but the meteors, which being bred of nothing else but of the vapors and exhalations sucked up by the Sun out of the earth, the Sea, and waters, yet are the same smoky vapors turned, and transformed into rain, snow, dew, rime, frost, and such like watery meteors, as by the contrary the rain clouds are often transformed and evaporated in blustering winds.

The second argument grounded on a show of reason is, that this filthy smoke, as well through the heat and strength thereof, as by a natural force and quality, is able and fit to purge both the head and stomach of rheums and distillations, as experience teaches, by the spitting and avoiding phlegm, immediately after the taking of it. But the fallacies of this Argument may easily appear, by my late preceding description of the meteors. For even as the smoky vapors sucked up by the sun, and stayed in the lowest and cold region of the air, are there contracted into clouds and turned into rain and such other watery meteors: So this stinking smoke being sucked up by the nose, and imprisoned in the cold and moist brains, is by their cold and wet faculties, turned and cast forth again in watery distillations, and so are you made free and purged of nothing, but that wherewith you willfully burdened yourselves: and therefore are you no wiser in taking tobacco for purging you of distillations, then if for preventing the colic you would take all kind of windy meats and drinks, and for preventing the Stone, you would take all kind of meats and drinks, that would breed gravel in the kidneys, and then when you were forced to avoid much wind out of your stomach, and much gravel in your urine, that you should attribute the thanks thereof to such nourishment as bred those within you, that caused this either to be expelled by the force of nature, or you to have burst at the broad side, as the Proverb is.

As for the other two reasons founded upon experience, the first of which is that the whole people would not have taken so general a good liking thereof, if they had not by experience found it very sovereign, and good for them: For an answer I say, how easily the minds of any people, wherewith God has replenished this world, may be drawn to the foolish affectation of any novelty, I leave it to the discreet judgment of any man that is reasonable.

Do we not daily see, that a man can no sooner bring over from beyond the Seas any new form of apparel, but that he cannot be thought a man of spirit, that would not presently imitate the same? And so from hand to hand it spreads, till it be practiced by all, not for any commodity that is in it, but only because it is come to be the fashion. For such is the force of that natural self love in every one of us, and such is the corruption of all, bred in the breast of everyone, as we cannot be content unless we imitate everything that our fellows do, and so prove ourselves capable of everything whereof they are capable, like Apes, counterfeiting the manners of others, to our own destruction. For let one or two of the greatest Masters of Mathematics in any of the two famous Universities, but constantly affirm any clear day, that they see some strange apparition in the skies: they will I warrant you be seconded by the greatest part of the students in that profession: So loath will they be, to be thought inferior to their fellows, either in depth of knowledge or sharpness of sight, and therefore the general good liking and embracing of this foolish custom, does but only proceed from that affectation of novelty, and popular error, whereof I have already spoken.

The other argument drawn from a mistaken experience, is but the more particular probation of this general idea, because it is alleged to be found true by proof, that by the taking of tobacco the masses do find themselves cured of various diseases as on the other part, no man ever received harm thereby. In this argument there is first a great mistaking and next a monstrous absurdity. For is it not a very great mistaking, to take *Non causam pro causa*, as they say in logic? because peradventure when a sick man has had his disease at the height, he has at that instant taken tobacco, and afterward his disease taking the natural course of declining, and consequently the patient of recovering his health, says, "the tobacco forsooth, was the worker of that miracle." Beside that, it is a thing well known to all Physicians, that the apprehension and conceit of the patient has by wakening and uniting the vital spirits, and so strengthening nature, a great power and virtue, to cure various diseases. For an evident proof of mistaking in these cases, I pray you; what foolish boy, what silly wench, what old doting wife, or ignorant country clown, is not a Physician for the toothache, for the colic, and various such common diseases? Yea, will not every man you meet withal, teach you a sundry cure for the same, and swear by that mean either himself, or some of his nearest kinsmen and friends was cured? And yet I hope no man is so

# A COUNTERBLAST TO TOBACCO

foolish as to believe them. And all these toys do only proceed from the mistaking *Non causam pro causa*, as I have already said, and so if a man chance to recover one of any disease, after he has taken tobacco, that must have the thanks of all. But by the contrary, if a man smokes himself to death with it (and many have done so) then some other disease must bear the blame for that fault. So do old harlots thank their prostitution for their many years, that custom being healthful (say they) *ad purgandos Renes*, but never have mind how many die of the pox in the flower of their youth. And so do old drunkards think they prolong their days, by their swinelike diet, but never remember how many die drowned in drink before they be middle aged.

And what greater absurdity can there be, then to say that one cure shall serve for various, nay, contrary manners of diseases? It is an undoubted ground among all Physicians, that there is almost no sort either of nourishment or medicine, that has not some thing in it disagreeable to some part of mans body, because, as I have already said, the nature of the temperature of every part, is so different from another, that according to the old Proverb, that which is good for the head, is evil for the neck and the shoulders. For even as a strong enemy, that invades a town or fortress, although in his siege thereof, he does besiege and surround it round about, yet he makes his breach and entry, at some one or few special parts thereof, which he has tried and found to be weakest and least able to resist; so sickness also makes her particular assault, upon such part or parts of our body, as are weakest and easiest to be overcome by that sort of disease, which then assails us, although all the rest of the body by sympathy feels itself, to be as it were belayed, and besieged by the affliction of that special part, the grief and smart thereof

# A COUNTERBLAST TO TOBACCO

being by the sense of feeling dispersed through all the rest of our members.

And therefore the skillful physician presses by such cures, to purge and strengthen that part which is afflicted, as are only fit for that sort of disease, and do best agree with the nature of that infirm part; which being abused to a disease of another nature, would prove as hurtful for the one, as helpful for the other. Yea, not only will a skillful and wary Physician be careful to use no cure but that which is fit for that sort of disease, but he will also consider all other circumstances, and make the remedies suitable thereunto; as the temperature of the clime where the patient is, the constitution of the Planets, the time of the Moon, the season of the year, the age and complexion of the patient, and the present state of his body, in strength or weakness. For one cure must not ever be used for the self-same disease, but according to the varying of any of the aforesaid circumstances, that sort of remedies must be used which are fittest for the same. Conversely, in this case, such is the miraculous omnipotence of our strong flavored tobacco, as it cures all sorts of diseases (which never any drug could do before) in all persons, and at all times. It cures all manner of infections, either in the head or stomach (if you believe their proclamations) although in very deed it both corrupts the brain, and by causing excessive digestion, fills the stomach full of crudities. It cures the gout in the feet, and (which is miraculous) in that very instant when the smoke thereof, as light, flies up into the head, the virtue thereof, as heavy, runs down to the little toe. It helps all sorts of Agues. It makes a man sober that was drunk. It refreshes a weary man, and yet makes a man hungry. Being taken when they go to bed, it makes one sleep soundly, and yet being taken when a man is sleepy and drowsy, it will, as they say, awaken his brain, and quicken his understanding. As for curing of the pox, it serves for that use but only among the poxy Indian slaves. Here in England, it is refined, and will not design to cure here any other then cleanly and gentlemanly diseases.

Omnipotent power of tobacco!

And if it could by the smoke thereof chase our devils, as the smoke of Tobias' fish did (which I am sure could smell no stronger) it would serve for a precious relic, both for the superstitious Priests, and the insolent Puritans, to cast out devils withal. Admitting then, and not confessing that the use thereof were healthful for some sorts of diseases; should it be used for all sicknesses? Should it be used by all men? Should it be used at all times? Yea should it be used by able, young, strong, healthful men? Medicine has that virtue that it never leaves a man in that state wherein it finds him; it makes a sick man whole, but a whole man sick. And as Medicine helps nature being taken at times of necessity, so being ever and continually used, it also will weaken, weary, and wear nature. What speak I of Medicine? Nay let a man every hour of the day, or as oft as many in this country use to take tobacco, let a man I say, but take as oft the best sorts of nourishment in meat and drink that can be devised, he shall with the continual use thereof weaken both his head and his stomach; all his members shall become feeble, his spirits dull, and in the end, as a drowsy, lazy belly-god, he shall vanish into a lethargic way.

And from this weakness it proceeds, that many in this kingdom have had such a continual use of taking this unsavory smoke, as now they are not able to forbear the same, no more than an old drunkard can abide to be long sober, without falling into an incurable weakness and evil constitution; for their continual custom has made them, *habitum, alteram naturam*- so to those that from their birth have been continually nourished upon poison and things venomous, wholesome meats are only a poison.

Thus having, as I trust, sufficiently answered the most principal arguments that are used in defense of this vile custom, it rests only to inform you what sins and vanities you commit in the filthy abuse thereof. First are you not guilty of sinful and shameful lust? (for lust may be as well in any of the senses as in feeling) that although you be troubled with no disease, but are in perfect health, yet can you neither be merry at a gathering, nor lascivious in the bed, if you lack tobacco to provoke your appetite to any of those sorts of recreation, lusting after it as the children of Israel did in the wilderness after Quails?

Secondly it is, as you use or rather abuse it, a branch of the sin of drunkenness, which is the root of all sins, for as the only delight that drunkards take in wine is in the strength of the taste, and the force of the fume thereof that mounts up to the brain, for no drunkards love any weak, or sweet drink, so are not those (I mean the strong heat and the fume), the only qualities that make tobacco so delectable to all the lovers of it? And as no man likes strong heady drink the first day (because *nemo repente fit turpissimus*), but by custom is piece and piece allured, while in the end, a drunkard will have as great a thirst with a draught as when he has need of it. So is not this the very case of all the great takers of tobacco? Which therefore they

# A COUNTERBLAST TO TOBACCO

themselves do attribute to a bewitching quality in it.

Thirdly, is it not the greatest sin of all, that you the people of all sorts of this Kingdom, who are created and ordained by God to bestow both your persons and goods for the maintenance both of the honor and safety of your King and Commonwealth, should disable yourselves in both? In your persons having by this continual vile custom brought yourselves to this shameful imbecility, that you are not able to ride or walk the journey of a Jews' Sabbath, but you must have a hot coal brought to you from the next poor house to kindle your tobacco with? Whereas he cannot be thought able for any service in the war, that cannot endure oftentimes the want of meat, drink, and sleep, much more then must he endure the want of tobacco.

In the times of the many glorious and victorious battles fought by this nation, there was no word of tobacco. But now if it were time of war, and that you were to make some sudden ambush upon your enemies, if any of you should seek leisure to stay behind his fellow for taking of tobacco, for my part I should never be sorry for any evil chance that might befall him. To take a custom in any thing that be left again, is most harmful to the people of any land. Decadence and delicacy were the wrack and overthrow, first of the Persian, and next of the Roman Empire. And this very custom of taking tobacco (whereof our present purpose is), is even at this day accounted so effeminate among the Indians themselves, as in the market they will offer no price for a slave to be sold, whom they find to be a great tobacco smoker.

Now how you are by this custom disabled in your goods,

let the gentry of this land bear witness, some of them bestowing three, some four hundred pounds a year upon this precious stink, which I am sure might be bestowed upon many far better uses. I read indeed of a knavish Courtier, who for abusing the favor of the Emperor Alexander Severus, his master, by taking bribes to intercede, for sundry persons in his master's ear (for whom he never once opened his mouth) was justly choked with smoke, with this doom, *Fumo pereat, qui fumum vendidit*: but of so many smokers, as are at this present in this kingdom, I never read nor heard.

And for the vanities committed in this filthy custom, is it not both great vanity and uncleanliness, that at the table, a place of respect, of cleanliness, of modesty, men should not be ashamed, to sit smoking Tobacco pipes, and puffing of the smoke of tobacco one to another, making the filthy smoke and stink thereof, to exhale next to the dishes, and infect the air, when very often, men that abhor it are at their repast? Surely Smoke becomes a kitchen far better then a dining chamber, and yet it makes a kitchen also oftentimes in the inward parts of men, soiling and infecting them, with an unctuous and oily kind of soot, as has been found in some great tobacco takers, that after their death were opened. And not only meat time, but no other time nor action is exempted from the public use of this uncivil trick: So as if the wives of Diepe list to contest with this nation for good manners their worst manners would in all reason be found at least not so dishonest (as ours are) in this point. The publikc use whereof, at all times, and in all places, has now so far prevailed, as various men very sound both in judgment, and complexion, have been at last forced to take it also without desire, partly because they were ashamed to seem singular (like

# A COUNTERBLAST TO TOBACCO

the two Philosophers that were forced to duck themselves in that rain water, and so become fools as well as the rest of the people) and partly, to be as one that was content to eat Garlic (which he did not love) that he might not be troubled with the smell of it, in the breath of his fellows.

And is it not a great vanity, that a man cannot heartily welcome his friend now, but with the immediate offer of tobacco? No it is become in place of a cure, a point of good fellowship, and he that will refuse to take a pipe of tobacco among his fellows, (though by his own election he would rather feel the savor of a sink) is accounted peevish and no good company, even as they do with drinking in the cold Eastern Countries.

Yea the Mistress cannot in a more mannerly kind, entertain her servant, then by giving him out of her fair hand a pipe of tobacco. But herein is not only a great vanity, but a great contempt of God's good gifts, that the sweetness of mans breath, being a good gift of God, should be willfully corrupted by this stinking smoke, wherein I must confess, it has too strong a virtue, and so that which is an ornament of nature, and can neither by any artifice be at the first acquired, nor once lost, be recovered again, shall be filthily corrupted with an incurable stink, which vile quality is as directly contrary to that wrong opinion which is held of the wholesomeness thereof, as the venom of putrefaction is contrary to the virtue of a Preservative.

Moreover, which is a great iniquity, and against all humanity, the husband shall not be ashamed, to reduce thereby his delicate, wholesome, and clean complexioned wife, to that

# A COUNTERBLAST TO TOBACCO

extreme, that either she must also corrupt her sweet breath therewith, or else resolve to live in a perpetual stinking torment.

Haue you not reason then to be ashamed, and to forbear this filthy behavior, so basely grounded, so foolishly received and so grossly mistaken in the right use thereof? In your abuse thereof sinning against God, harming yourselves both in persons and goods, and taking also thereby the marks and notes of vanity upon you, by the custom thereof making yourselves to be wondered at by all foreign and civil nations, and by all strangers that come among you, to be scorned and condemned. A custom loathsome to the eye, hateful to the nose, harmful to the brain, dangerous to the lungs, and in the black stinking fume thereof, nearest resembling the horrible Stygian smoke of the pit that is bottomless.

**THE END**

# A COUNTERBLAST TO TOBACCO

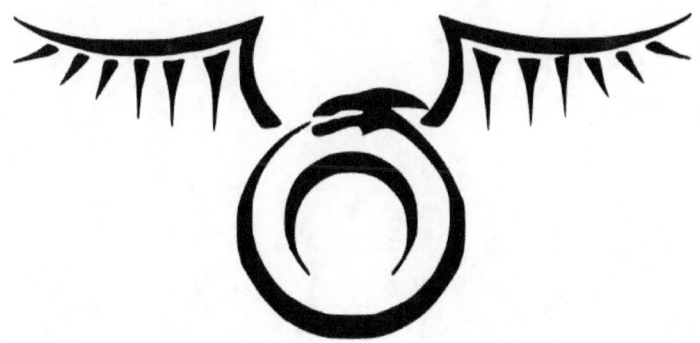

*It is the editors' fervent wish that those addicted to tobacco will seek cessation- an attempt I, the editor, am making as of the finalizing of this document to be released.*

*For those interested in the writings of King James, I have fully edited and modernized an edition of his "Daemonologie" ISBN 978-1537015798.*

www.ingramcontent.com/pod-product-compliance
Lightning Source LLC
Chambersburg PA
CBHW061454180526
45170CB00004B/1705